The Essential 5-Ingredient Keto Diet

Low-Carb, High-Fat Keto-Friendly 5-Ingredient Recipes

Dr. Marta Cox

TABLE OF CONTENTS

BREAKFAST RECIPES

Cheesy Ham Souffle

Serves: 4 Prep Time: 30 mins

Ingredients

- 1 cup cheddar cheese, shredded
- ½ cup heavy cream
- 6 large eggs
- 6 ounces ham, diced
- Salt and black pepper, to taste

Directions

1. Preheat the oven to 3500F and grease 4 ramekins gently.
2. Whisk together eggs in a medium bowl and add all other ingredients.
3. Mix well and pour the mixture into the ramekins.
4. Transfer into the ramekins and bake for about 18 minutes.
5. Remove from the oven and allow to slightly cool and serve.

Nutrition Amount per serving

Calories 342

Total Fat 26g 33%

Saturated Fat 13g 65%

Cholesterol 353mg 118%

Sodium 841mg 37%

Total Carbohydrate 3g 1%

Dietary Fiber 0.6g 2%

Total Sugars 0.8g

Protein 23.8g

Keto Breakfast Wrap

Serves: 1

Prep Time: 20 mins Ingredients

- 1 organic nori sheet
- 1½ avocado, sliced
- 3 pastured eggs

Total Sugars 0g

- ¼ teaspoon salt
- ½ tablespoon butter

Directions

1. Whisk eggs and salt in a bowl until combined.
2. Heat butter on medium heat in a frying pan and stir in whisked eggs.
3. Cook for about 3 minutes on both sides and dish out.
4. Place the omelet on top of the nori sheet and top with avocado slices.
5. Roll up the breakfast wrap and slice in half to serve.

Nutrition Amount per serving

Calories 476

Total Fat 38.8g 50%

Saturated Fat 12.2g 61%

Cholesterol 660mg 220%

Sodium 788mg 34%

Total Carbohydrate 11.7g 4%

Dietary Fiber 7.7g 28%

Total Sugars 0.5g

Protein 21g

Egg Crepes with Avocados

Serves: 2

Prep Time: 15 mins

Ingredients

- 4 eggs
- ¾ avocado, thinly sliced
- 2 teaspoons olive oil
- ½ cup alfalfa sprouts
- 4 slices turkey breast cold cuts, shredded

Directions

1. Heat olive oil over medium heat in a pan and crack in the eggs.
2. Spread the eggs lightly with the spatula and cook for about 3 minutes on both sides.
3. Dish out the egg crepe and top with turkey breast, alfalfa sprouts and avocado.
4. Roll up tightly and serve warm.

Nutrition Amount per serving Calories 372

Total Fat 25.9g 33% Saturated Fat 6g 30% Cholesterol 364mg

121%

Sodium 1000mg 43%

Breakfast Bacon Muffins

Serves: 6

Prep Time: 30 mins Ingredients

- 1 cup bacon bits
- 3 cups almond flour, organic
- ½ cup ghee, melted

Total Carbohydrate 9.3g 3% Dietary Fiber 4.4g 16% Total Sugars

4g

Protein 27.2g

- 1 teaspoon baking soda
- 4 eggs

Directions

1. Preheat the oven to 3500F and line muffin tins with muffin liners.
2. Melt ghee in a bowl and stir in the almond flour and baking soda.
3. Mix well and add the bacon bits and eggs.
4. Divide the mixture into the muffin tins and transfer into the oven.
5. Bake for about 20 minutes and remove from the oven to serve.

Nutrition Amount per serving

Calories 485

Total Fat 49.8g 64% Saturated Fat 37.3g 186% Cholesterol

156mg 52% Sodium 343mg 15%

Keto Non-Oatmeal Breakfast

Serves: 2

Prep Time: 25 mins Ingredients

Total Carbohydrate 6.9g 3% Dietary Fiber 2.6g 9%

Total Sugars 4.2g Protein 7.7g

- 1 cup organic coconut milk, full-fat
- 1 cup cauliflower, riced
- 1/3 cup fresh organic raspberries
- 3 drops liquid Stevia
- 3 tablespoons unsweetened coconut, shredded

Directions

1. Mix together cauliflower and coconut milk and pour in a pot.
2. Cook over medium heat until cauliflower warms up and add raspberries.
3. Mash the raspberries and stir in coconut and Stevia.
4. Cover the lid and cook for about 10 minutes.
5. Dish into a bowl and serve warm.

Nutrition Amount per serving

Calories 326

Total Fat 31.3g 40%

Saturated Fat 27.6g 138%

Cholesterol 0mg 0%

Protein 4.3g
Sodium 35mg 2%

Total Carbohydrate 12.9g 5%

Dietary Fiber 5.9g 21%

Total Sugars 6.6g

Spaghetti Squash Hash Browns

Serves: 3

Prep Time: 25 mins

Ingredients

- Sea salt and black pepper, to taste
- 1½ cups spaghetti squash
- 3 tablespoons avocado oil, for frying
- ½ cup sour cream
- ½ cup green onions

Directions

1. Season the spaghetti squash with sea salt and black pepper.
2. Add green onions and sour cream and form into patties.
3. Heat avocado oil in a skillet over medium heat and add patties.
4. Fry until golden brown from both sides and dish out to serve.

Nutrition Amount per serving

Calories 122

Total Fat 10.1g 13% Saturated Fat 5.4g 27% Cholesterol 17mg

6%

Sodium 32mg 1%

Total Carbohydrate 7.1g 3%

Mini Bacon Guacamole Cups

Dietary Fiber 1g 4% Total Sugars 0.5g

Serves: 4 Prep Time: 40 mins

Ingredients

- 1 ripe avocado
- 9 bacon slices, 6 slices halved, and 3 slices quartered
- 2 tablespoons onion, minced
- Kosher salt and black pepper, to taste
- 1 small jalapeno, seeded and minced

Directions

1. Preheat the oven to 4000F and turn 4 mini-muffin pans upside down on a baking sheet.
2. Spray the tops of the overturned muffin tins and place the quarter of the slice on top.
3. Wrap the sides of the mini-muffin pans with the longer portions of bacon and secure with a toothpick.
4. Bake for about 25 minutes and remove carefully from the mini muffin cups.
5. Meanwhile, mash avocado with a fork in a medium bowl and stir in the jalapeno, onions, salt and black pepper.
6. Put the guacamole in the bacon cups and serve warm.

Nutrition Amount per serving

Calories 337

Total Fat 27.7g 36%

Saturated Fat 7.9g 40%

Cholesterol 47mg 16%

Sodium 991mg 43%

Total Carbohydrate 5.6g 2%

Dietary Fiber 3.6g 13%

Total Sugars 0.6g

Protein 16.9g

Coconut Macadamia Bars

Serves: 6

Prep Time: 10 mins

Ingredients

- ¼ cup coconut oil
- 10 drops Stevia drops
- 60 grams macadamia nuts, crushed
- ½ cup almond butter
- 6 tablespoons unsweetened coconut, shredded

Directions

1. Mix together coconut oil, almond butter and coconut in a bowl.
2. Stir in Stevia and macadamia nuts and mix well.
3. Pour this mixture into a baking dish and refrigerate overnight.
4. Slice and serve chilled.

Nutrition Amount per serving

Calories 176

Total Fat 19.1g 24%

Saturated Fat 10.6g 53%

Cholesterol 0mg 0%

Sodium 2mg 0%

Total Carbohydrate 2.4g 1%

Dietary Fiber 1.4g 5%

Total Sugars 0.8g

Protein 1.2g

Avocado and Smoked Salmon Omelet

Serves: 2

Prep Time: 15 mins

Ingredients

- 4 large eggs
- 3 teaspoons extra virgin olive oil, divided
- 2 ounce smoked salmon
- Pinch of salt
- ½ avocado, sliced

Directions

1. Whisk together eggs and salt in a bowl.
2. Heat 2 teaspoons of oil over medium heat in a skillet and stir in the egg mixture.
3. Cook for about 2 minutes until the center is still a bit runny and the bottom is set.
4. Flip the omelet and cook for about 30 seconds.
5. Transfer to a plate and top with smoked salmon and avocado
6. Sprinkle with the remaining olive oil and serve.

Nutrition Amount per serving

Calories 339

Total Fat 28g 36%

Saturated Fat 6.4g 32%

Cholesterol 379mg 126%

Sodium 865mg 38%

Total Carbohydrate 5.1g 2%

Dietary Fiber 3.4g 12%

Total Sugars 1g

Protein 18.7g

Banana Pancakes

Serves: 4

Prep Time: 25 mins

Ingredients

- 1 medium banana
- 2 large eggs
- 2 tablespoons butter
- 1 tablespoon sugar free maple syrup
- 4 tablespoons ricotta cheese

Directions

1. Put the banana and eggs in a blender and blend until smooth.
2. Heat ½ tablespoon of butter over medium heat in a large nonstick pan and pour 2 tablespoons of the batter.
3. Cook for about 2 minutes until bubbles appear on the surface.
4. Flip the pancakes gently with a spatula and cook for 2 more minutes.
5. Dish out the pancakes to a plate and repeat with the remaining batter.

Nutrition Amount per serving

Calories 147

Total Fat 9.6g 12%

Saturated Fat 5.2g 26%

Cholesterol 113mg 38%

Sodium 96mg 4%

Total Carbohydrate 11.1g 4%

Dietary Fiber 0.8g 3%

Total Sugars 6.8g

Protein 5.3g

Clementine and Pistachio Ricotta

Serves: 1

Prep Time: 10 mins

Ingredients

- 2 teaspoons pistachios, chopped
- ⅓ cup ricotta
- 2 strawberries
- 1 tablespoon butter, melted
- 1 clementine, peeled and segmented

Directions

1. Put the ricotta into a serving bowl.
2. Top with clementine segments, strawberries, pistachios and butter to serve.

Nutrition Amount per serving

Calories 311

Total Fat 25.1g 32%

Saturated Fat 15.1g 76%

Cholesterol 71mg 24%

Sodium 243mg 11%

Total Carbohydrate 12.7g 5%

Dietary Fiber 1.2g 4%

Total Sugars 7.1g

Protein 10.7g

APPETIZERS AND DESSERTS

Caprese Snack

Serves: 4

Prep Time: 5 mins

Ingredients

- 8 oz. mozzarella, mini cheese balls
- 8 oz. cherry tomatoes
- 2 tablespoons green pesto
- Salt and black pepper, to taste
- 1 tablespoon garlic powder

Directions

1. Slice the mozzarella balls and tomatoes in half.
2. Stir in the green pesto and season with garlic powder, salt and pepper to serve.

Nutrition Amount per serving

Calories 407

Total Fat 34.5g 44%

Saturated Fat 7.4g 37%

Cholesterol 30mg 10%

Sodium 343mg 15%

Total Carbohydrate 6.3g 2%

Dietary Fiber 0.9g 3%

Total Sugars 2g

Protein 19.4g

Almond Flour Crackers

Serves: 6

Prep Time: 25 mins

Ingredients

- 2 tablespoons sunflower seeds
- 1 cup almond flour
- ¾ teaspoon sea salt
- 1 tablespoon whole psyllium husks
- 1 tablespoon coconut oil

Directions

1. Preheat the oven to 3500F and grease a baking sheet lightly.
2. Mix together sunflower seeds, almond flour, sea salt, coconut oil, psyllium husks and 2 tablespoons of water in a bowl.
3. Transfer into a blender and blend until smooth.
4. Form a dough out of this mixture and roll it on the parchment paper until 1/16 inch thick.
5. Slice into 1 inch squares and season with some sea salt.
6. Arrange the squares on the baking sheet and transfer to the oven.
7. Bake for about 15 minutes until edges are crisp and brown.
8. Allow to cool and separate into squares to serve.

Nutrition Amount per serving

Calories 141

Total Fat 11.6g 15%

Saturated Fat 2.7g 13%

Cholesterol 0mg 0%

Sodium 241mg 10%

Total Carbohydrate 5.2g 2%

Dietary Fiber 3.1g 11%

Total Sugars 0g

Protein 4.2g

Crispy Baked Zucchini Fries

Serves: 4

Prep Time: 30 mins

Ingredients

- ¾ cup parmesan cheese, grated
- 2 medium zucchinis, chopped into small sticks
- 1 large egg
- ¼ teaspoon black pepper
- ¼ teaspoon garlic powder

Directions

1. Preheat the oven to 4250F and grease a baking sheet lightly.
2. Whisk egg in one bowl and mix together parmesan cheese, black pepper and garlic powder in another bowl.
3. Dip each zucchini stick in the egg and then dredge in the dry mixture.
4. Transfer to the baking sheet and place in the oven.
5. Bake for about 20 minutes until golden and broil for 3 minutes to serve.

Nutrition Amount per serving

Calories 102
Total Fat 5.9g 8%
Saturated Fat 3.4g 17%
Cholesterol 62mg 21%
Sodium 222mg 10%

Total Carbohydrate 4.3g 2%
Dietary Fiber 1.1g 4%
Total Sugars 1.8g
Protein 9.6g

Low Carb Onion Rings

Serves: 6

Prep Time: 30 mins

Ingredients

- 2 medium white onions, sliced into ½ inch thick rings
- ½ cup coconut flour
- 4 large eggs
- 4 oz pork rinds
- 1 cup parmesan cheese, grated

Directions

1. Preheat an Air fryer to 3900F and grease a fryer basket.
2. Put coconut flour in one bowl, eggs in the second bowl and pork rinds and parmesan cheese in the third bowl.
3. Coat the onion rings through the three bowls one by one and repeat.
4. Place the coated onion rings in the fryer basket and cook for about 15 minutes.
5. Dish out to a platter and serve with your favorite low carb sauce.

Nutrition Amount per serving

Calories 270

Total Fat 15.1g 19%

Saturated Fat 7.1g 35%

Cholesterol 164mg 55%

Sodium 586mg 25%

Total Carbohydrate 11g 4%

Dietary Fiber 4.8g 17% Total

Sugars 1.8g Protein 24.1g

Broccoli Fritters with Cheddar Cheese

Serves: 4

Prep Time: 20 mins

Ingredients

- 1 cup cheddar cheese, shredded
- 8 ounces broccoli, chopped, steamed and drained
- 2 large eggs, beaten
- 1 tablespoon avocado oil
- 2 tablespoons oat fiber

Directions

1. Mix together broccoli with cheddar cheese, eggs and oat fiber in a bowl.
2. Heat avocado oil over medium heat in a nonstick pan and add the broccoli mixture in small chunks.
3. Cook for about 5 minutes on both sides until browned and dish onto a platter to serve.

Nutrition Amount per serving

Calories 178

Total Fat 12.6g 16%

Saturated Fat 6.8g 34%

Cholesterol 123mg 41%

Sodium 236mg 10%

Total Carbohydrate 5.3g 2%

Dietary Fiber 2g 7%

Total Sugars 1.4g

Protein 12.1g

Cheesy Low Carb Creamed Spinach

Serves: 8

Prep Time: 25 mins

Ingredients

- 2 (10 oz) packages frozen chopped spinach, thawed
- 3 tablespoons butter
- 6 ounces cream cheese
- Onion powder, salt and black pepper
- ½ cup parmesan cheese, grated

Directions

1. Mix together 2 tablespoons of butter with cream cheese, parmesan cheese, salt and black pepper in a bowl.
2. Heat the rest of the butter on medium heat in a small pan and add onion powder.
3. Sauté for about 1 minute and add spinach.
4. Cover and cook on low heat for about 5 minutes.
5. Stir in the cheese mixture and cook for about 3 minutes.
6. Dish into a bowl and serve hot.

Nutrition Amount per serving

Calories 141

Total Fat 12.8g 16%
Saturated Fat 8g 40%

Cholesterol 37mg 12%

Sodium 182mg 8%

Total Carbohydrate 3.5g 1%

Dietary Fiber 1.6g 6%
Total Sugars 0.5g

Protein 4.8g

Jicama Fries

Serves: 2

Prep Time: 20 mins

Ingredients

- 2 tablespoons avocado oil
- 1 Jicama, cut into fries
- 1 tablespoon garlic powder
- ½ cup parmesan cheese, grated
- Salt and black pepper, to taste

Directions

1. Preheat the Air fryer to 4000F and grease the fryer basket.
2. Boil jicama fries for about 10 minutes and drain well.
3. Mix jicama fries with garlic powder, salt and black pepper in a bowl.
4. Place in the fryer basket and cook for about 10 minutes.
5. Dish onto a platter and serve warm.

Spicy Tuna Rolls

Serves: 2

Prep Time: 15 mins

Ingredients

- 1 pouch StarKist Selects E.V.O.O. Wild Caught Yellowfin Tuna
- 1 medium cucumber, thinly sliced lengthwise
- 1 teaspoon hot sauce
- 2 slices avocado, diced
- Cayenne, salt and black pepper

Directions

1. Mix together tuna with hot sauce, cayenne, salt and black pepper in a bowl until combined.
2. Put the tuna mixture on the cucumber slices and top with avocado.
3. Roll up the cucumber and secure with 2 toothpicks to serve.

Nutrition Amount per serving

Calories 139	Sodium 86mg 4%
Total Fat 6.5g 8%	Total Carbohydrate 8.4g 3%
Saturated Fat 1.2g 6%	Dietary Fiber 2.9g 10%
Cholesterol 22mg 7%	Total Sugars 2.8

PORK AND BEEF RECIPES

Keto Burger Fat Bombs

Serves: 10

Prep Time: 30 mins

Ingredients

- ½ teaspoon garlic powder
- 1 pound ground beef
- Kosher salt and black pepper, to taste
- ¼ (8 oz.) block cheddar cheese, cut into 20 pieces
- 2 tablespoons cold butter, cut into 20 pieces

Directions

1. Preheat the oven to 3750F and grease mini muffin tins with cooking spray.
2. Season the beef with garlic powder, kosher salt and black pepper in a medium bowl.
3. Press about 1 tablespoon of beef into each muffin tin, covering the bottom completely.
4. Layer with small piece of butter and add 1 more tablespoon of beef.
5. Top with a piece of cheese in each cup and press the remaining beef.
6. Transfer to the oven and bake for about 20 minutes.
7. Allow to slightly cool and dish out to serve hot.

Nutrition Amount per serving

Calories 128

Total Fat 7g 9%

Saturated Fat 3.7g 19%

Cholesterol 53mg 18%

Sodium 81mg 4%

Total Carbohydrate 0.2g 0%

Dietary Fiber 0g 0%

Total Sugars 0.1g

Protein 15.2g

Ice-Burgers

Serves: 4

Prep Time: 30 mins

Ingredients

- 4 slices bacon, cooked and crisped
- 1 large head iceberg lettuce, sliced into 8 rounds
- 1 pound ground beef
- 4 slices cheddar cheese
- Kosher salt and black pepper, to taste

Directions

1. Make 4 large patties out of ground beef and season both sides with salt and black pepper.
2. Grill for about 10 minutes per side and top with cheddar cheese slices.
3. Place one iceberg round on a plate and layer with grilled beef.
4. Place a slice of bacon and close with second iceberg round.
5. Repeat with the remaining ingredients and serve warm.

Nutrition Amount per serving
Calories 452

Total Fat 24.6g 32% Saturated Fat 11.2g 56% Cholesterol 152mg

51%

Sodium 698mg 30%
Total Carbohydrate 6.3g 2% Dietary Fiber 1.2g 4%

Total Sugars 2g Protein 49.3g

Jamaican Jerk Pork Roast

Serves: 3

Prep Time: 35 mins

Ingredients

- 1 tablespoon butter
- 1/8 cup beef broth
- 1 pound pork shoulder
- 1/8 cup Jamaican jerk spice blend
- Salt, to taste

Directions

1. Season the pork with Jamaican jerk spice blend.
2. Heat the butter in the pot and add seasoned pork.
3. Cook for about 5 minutes and add beef broth.
4. Cover with lid and cook for about 20 minutes on low heat.
5. Dish out on a serving platter and serve hot.

Nutrition Amount per serving

Calories 477

Total Fat 36.2g 46%

Protein 35.4g

Saturated Fat 14.3g 72%

Cholesterol 146mg 49%

Sodium 212mg 9%

Total Carbohydrate 0g 0%
Dietary Fiber 0g 0%Total
Sugars 0g

Pork Carnitas

Serves: 3

Prep Time: 40 mins

Ingredients

- 1 pound pork shoulder, bone-in
- Salt and black pepper, to taste
- 1 tablespoon butter
- 1 orange, juiced
- ½ teaspoon garlic powder

Directions

1. Season the pork with salt and black pepper.
2. Put butter in the pressure cooker and add garlic powder.
3. Sauté for 1 minute and add seasoned pork.
4. Sauté for 3 minutes and pour orange juice.
5. Lock the lid and cook on high pressure for about 20 minutes.
6. Naturally release the pressure and dish out.
7. Shred the pork with a fork and transfer back to the cooker.
8. Sauté for about 3 minutes and serve warm.

Nutrition Amount per serving

Calories 506

Total Fat 36.3g 46%

Saturated Fat 14.3g 72%

Cholesterol 146mg 49%

Sodium 130mg 6%

Total Carbohydrate 7.6g 3%

Dietary Fiber 1.5g 5%

Total Sugars 5.8g

Protein 35.9g

Zesty Pork Chops

Serves: 4

Prep Time: 50 mins

Ingredients

- 4 tablespoons butter
- 3 tablespoons lemon juice
- 4 pork chops, bone-in
- 2 tablespoons low carb flour mix
- 1 cup picante sauce

Directions

1. Coat the pork chops with low carb flour mix.
2. Mix picante sauce and lemon juice in a bowl.
3. Heat oil in a skillet on medium heat and add the chops and picante mixture.
4. Cook covered for about 35 minutes and dish out to serve hot.

Nutrition Amount per serving

Calories 398 Total Fat 33.4g 43%
Saturated Fat 15g 75% Cholesterol 99mg 33%

Sodium 441mg 19%

Total Carbohydrate 4g 1%
Dietary Fiber 0.7g 3% Total Sugars 2.1g Protein 19.7g

Greek Pork Gyros

Serves: 4

Prep Time: 40 mins

Ingredients

- 4 garlic cloves
- 3 teaspoons ground marjoram
- 1 pound pork meat, ground
- Salt and black pepper, to taste
- ½ small onion, chopped

Directions

1. Preheat the oven to 4000F and grease a loaf pan lightly.
2. Put onions, garlic, marjoram, salt and black pepper in a food processor and process until well combined.
3. Add ground pork meat and process again.
4. Press meat mixture into the loaf pan until compact and very tight.
5. Tightly cover with tin foil and poke some holes in the foil.
6. Bake in the oven for about 25 minutes and dish out to serve warm.

Nutrition Amount per serving

Calories 310

Total Fat 24.2g 31% Saturated Fat 9g 45% Cholesterol 80mg

27%

Total Sugars 0.4g Protein 19.4g Sodium 66mg 3%

Total Carbohydrate 2.1g 1% Dietary Fiber 0.4g 2%

Garlic Rosemary Pork Chops

Serves: 4

Prep Time: 30 mins Ingredients

- 1 tablespoon rosemary, freshly minced
- 2 garlic cloves, minced
- 4 pork loin chops
- ½ cup butter, melted
- Salt and black pepper, to taste

Directions

1. Preheat the oven to 3750F and season pork chops with salt and black pepper.
2. Mix together ¼ cup butter, rosemary and garlic in a small bowl.
3. Heat the rest of the butter in an oven safe skillet and add pork chops.
4. Sear for about 4 minutes per side until golden and brush pork chops generously with garlic butter.
5. Place skillet in the oven and bake for about 15 minutes until cooked through.
6. Dish out and serve hot.

Nutrition Amount per serving

Calories 465

Total Fat 43g 55%

Saturated Fat 22.1g 110%

Cholesterol 130mg 43%

Sodium 220mg 10%

Total Carbohydrate 1.1g 0%

Dietary Fiber 0.4g 1%

Total Sugars 0g

Protein 18.4g

Lemony Grilled Pork Chops

Serves: 4

Prep Time: 20 mins

Ingredients

- 2 tablespoons extra-virgin olive oil
- 4 pork chops
- 2 tablespoons butter
- Kosher salt and black pepper, to taste
- 2 lemons, sliced

Directions

1. Preheat the grill to high heat.
2. Brush pork chops with olive oil and season with salt and black pepper.
3. Put the pork chops on grill and top with lemon slices.
4. Grill for about 10 minutes per side until lemons are charred and chops are cooked through.
5. Dish out on a platter and serve hot.

Nutrition Amount per serving

Calories 375

Total Fat 32.7g 42%

Saturated Fat 12.1g 61%

Cholesterol 84mg 28%

Sodium 97mg 4%

Total Carbohydrate 2.7g 1%

Dietary Fiber 0.8g 3%

Total Sugars 0.7g

Protein 18.4g

Cheddar Maple Squash

Serves: 4

Prep Time: 30 mins

Ingredients

- 1½ pounds summer squash, peeled, halved, seeded, and cut into 1½ inch cubes
- 1 cup aged white cheddar cheese, coarsely grated
- 1 tablespoon sugar free maple syrup
- 1 tablespoon fresh sage, chopped and crushed
- 2 slices pork bacon, cooked and chopped

Directions

1. Boil the summer squash for about 15 minutes and mash with a potato masher.
2. Stir in cheddar cheese, sage and maple syrup and top with cooked pork bacon to serve.

Nutrition Amount per serving

Calories 196

Total Fat 13.7g 18%

Saturated Fat 7.4g 37%

Cholesterol 40mg 13%

Sodium 414mg 18%

Total Carbohydrate 7.1g 3%

Dietary Fiber 2.1g 7%

Total Sugars 3.1g

Protein 12.7g

Spinach Pork Roll Ups

Serves: 8

Prep Time: 15 mins

Ingredients

- 2 teaspoons honey mustard
- 8 thin slices bacon, smoked
- 1 cup Monterey Jack cheese, cut lengthwise into quarters
- 1 cup fresh baby spinach leaves
- ½ medium red bell pepper, seeded and cut into thin strips

Directions

1. Spread the honey mustard over bacon slices.
2. Divide spinach leaves among 8 plates and place bacon slices on it.
3. Top with red bell pepper and cheese to serve.

Nutrition Amount per serving

Calories 161

Total Fat 12.3g 16%

Saturated Fat 5.3g 27%

Cholesterol 33mg 11%

Sodium 524mg 23%

Total Carbohydrate 1.6g 1%

Dietary Fiber 0.2g 1%

Total Sugars 0.7g

Protein 10.7g

Stuffed Pork Chops

Serves: 6

Prep Time: 40 mins

Ingredients

- 4 garlic cloves, minced
- 2 pounds cut boneless pork chops
- 1½ teaspoons salt
- 8 oz. provolone cheese
- 2 cups baby spinach

Directions

1. Preheat the oven to 3500F and grease a baking sheet
2. Mix garlic with salt and rub on one side of the pork chops.
3. Place half of the pork chops garlic side down on a baking sheet and top with spinach and provolone cheese.
4. Top with rest of the pork chops garlic side up and place in the oven.
5. Bake for about 30 minutes and dish out to serve hot.

Nutrition Amount per serving

Calories 430

Total Fat 20.2g 26%

Saturated Fat 9.8g 49%

Cholesterol 165mg 55%

Sodium 1005mg 44%

Total Carbohydrate 1.8g 1%

Dietary Fiber 0.3g 1%

Total Sugars 0.3g

Protein 57.2g

Pork with Butternut Squash Stew

Serves: 4

Prep Time: 40 mins

Ingredients

- ½ pound butternut squash, peeled and cubed
- 1 pound lean pork
- 2 tablespoons butter
- Salt and black pepper, to taste
- 1 cup beef stock

Directions

1. Put the butter and lean pork in a skillet and cook for about 5 minutes.
2. Add butternut squash, beef stock and season with salt and black pepper.
3. Cover with lid and cook for about 25 minutes on medium low heat.
4. Dish out to a bowl and serve hot.

Nutrition Amount per serving

Calories 319

Total Fat 17.1g 22%

Saturated Fat 7.9g 39%

Cholesterol 105mg 35%

Sodium 311mg 14%

Total Carbohydrate 6.7g 2%

Dietary Fiber 1.1g 4%

Total Sugars 1.3g

Protein 33.7g

Keto Taco Casserole

Serves: 8

Prep Time: 55 mins

Ingredients

- 2 pounds ground beef
- 1 tablespoon extra-virgin olive oil
- Taco seasoning mix, kosher salt and black pepper
- 2 cups Mexican cheese, shredded
- 6 large eggs, lightly beaten

Directions

2. Preheat the oven to 3600F and grease a 2 quart baking dish.
3. Heat oil over medium heat in a large skillet and add ground beef.
4. Season with taco seasoning mix, kosher salt and black pepper.
5. Cook for about 5 minutes on each side and dish out to let cool slightly.
6. Whisk together eggs in the beef mixture and transfer the mixture to the baking dish.
7. Top with Mexican cheese and bake for about 25 minutes until set.
8. Remove from the oven and serve warm.

Nutrition Amount per serving

Calories 382

Total Fat 21.6g 28%

Saturated Fat 9.1g 45%

Cholesterol 266mg 89%

Sodium 363mg 16%

Total Carbohydrate 1.7g 1%

Dietary Fiber 0g 0%

Total Sugars 0.4g

Protein 45.3g

SEAFOOD RECIPES

Garlic Butter Salmon

Serves: 8

Prep Time: 40 mins Ingredients

- Kosher salt and black pepper, to taste
- 1 pound (3 pounds) salmon fillet, skin removed
- 4 tablespoons butter, melted
- 2 garlic cloves, minced
- ¼ cup parmesan cheese, freshly grated

Directions

1. Preheat the oven to 3500F and lightly grease a large baking sheet.

Calories 172

Total Fat 12.3g 16% Saturated Fat 6.2g 31%

2. eason the salmon with salt and black pepper and transfer to the baking sheet.
3. Mix together butter, garlic and parmesan cheese in a small bowl.
4. Marinate salmon in this mixture for about 1 hour.
5. Transfer to the oven and bake for about 25 minutes.
6. Additionally, broil for about 2 minutes until top becomes lightly golden.
7. Dish out onto a platter and serve hot.

Nutrition Amount per serving
Cholesterol 50mg 17%

Sodium 196mg 9%

Total Carbohydrate 0.8g 0%
Dietary Fiber 0g 0% Total Sugars 0g

Protein 15.6g

Tuscan Butter Salmon

Serves: 4

Prep Time: 35 mins

Ingredients

- 4 (6 oz) salmon fillets, patted dry with paper towels
- 3 tablespoons butter
- ¾ cup heavy cream
- Kosher salt and black pepper
- 2 cups baby spinach

Directions

1. Season the salmon with salt and black pepper.
2. Heat 1½ tablespoons butter over medium high heat in a large skillet and add salmon skin side up.
3. Cook for about 10 minutes on both sides until deeply golden and dish out onto a plate.
4. Heat the rest of the butter in the skillet and add spinach.
5. Cook for about 5 minutes and stir in the heavy cream.
6. Reduce heat to low and simmer for about 3 minutes.
7. Return the salmon to the skillet and mix well with the sauce.
8. Allow to simmer for about 3 minutes until salmon is cooked through.
9. Dish out and serve hot.

Nutrition Amount per serving

Calories 382

Total Fat 27.5g 35%

Saturated Fat 12.2g 61%

Cholesterol 129mg 43%

Sodium 157mg 7%

Total Carbohydrate 1.2g 0%

Dietary Fiber 0.3g 1%

Total Sugars 0.1g

Protein 34g

Mahi Mahi Stew

Serves: 3

Prep Time: 45 mins

Ingredients

- 2 tablespoons butter
- 2 pounds Mahi Mahi fillets, cubed
- 1 onion, chopped
- Salt and black pepper, to taste
- 2 cups homemade fish broth

Directions

1. Season the Mahi Mahi fillets with salt and black pepper.
2. Heat butter in a pressure cooker and add onion.
3. Sauté for about 3 minutes and stir in the seasoned Mahi Mahi fillets and fish broth.
4. Lock the lid and cook on High Pressure for about 30 minutes.
5. Naturally release the pressure and dish out to serve hot.

Nutrition Amount per serving

Calories 398

Total Fat 12.5g 16% Saturated Fat 6.4g 32% Cholesterol 290mg

97%

Sodium 803mg 35% Total Carbohydrate 5.5g 2% Dietary Fiber

1.5g 5%

Total Sugars 2.2g Protein 62.3g

Sour Cream Tilapia

Serves: 3

Prep Time: 3 hours 10 mins Ingredients

- ¾ cup homemade chicken broth
- 1 pound tilapia fillets
- 1 cup sour cream
- Salt and black pepper, to taste
- 1 teaspoon cayenne pepper

Directions

1. Put tilapia fillets in the slow cooker along with rest of the ingredients.
2. Cover the lid and cook on low for about 3 hours.
3. Dish out and serve hot.

Nutrition Amount per serving

Calories 300

Total Fat 17.9g 23%

Saturated Fat 10.7g 54%

Cholesterol 107mg 36%

Sodium 285mg 12%

Total Carbohydrate 3.9g 1%

Dietary Fiber 0.2g 1%

Total Sugars 0.4g

Protein 31.8g

Tilapia with Herbed Butter

Serves: 6

Prep Time: 35 mins

Ingredients

- 2 pounds tilapia fillets
- 12 garlic cloves, chopped finely
- 6 green broccoli, chopped
- 2 cups herbed butter
- Salt and black pepper, to taste

Directions

1. Season the tilapia fillets with salt and black pepper.
2. Put the seasoned tilapia along with all other ingredients in an Instant Pot and mix well.
3. Cover the lid and cook on High Pressure for about 25 minutes.
4. Dish out in a platter and serve hot.

Nutrition Amount per serving

Calories 281

Total Fat 10.4g 13%

Saturated Fat 4.3g 21%

Cholesterol 109mg 36%

Sodium 178mg 8%

Total Carbohydrate 9g 3%

Dietary Fiber 2.5g 9%

Total Sugars 1.9g

Protein 38.7g

Roasted Trout

Serves: 4

- ½ cup fresh lemon juice
- 1 pound trout fish fillets
- 4 tablespoons butter
- Salt and black pepper, to taste
- 1 teaspoon dried rosemary, crushed

Directions

1. Put ½ pound trout fillets in a dish and sprinkle with lemon juice and dried rosemary.
2. Season with salt and black pepper and transfer into a skillet.
3. Add butter and cook, covered on medium low heat for about 35 minutes.
4. Dish out the fillets in a platter and serve with a sauce.

Nutrition Amount per serving

Calories 349

Total Fat 28.2g 36%

Saturated Fat 11.7g 58%

Cholesterol 31mg 10%

Sodium 88mg 4%

Total Carbohydrate 1.1g 0%

Dietary Fiber 0.3g 1%

Total Sugars 0.9g

Protein 23.3g

Sour Fish with Herbed Butter

Serves: 3

- 2 tablespoons herbed butter
- 3 cod fillets
- 1 tablespoon vinegar
- Salt and black pepper, to taste
- ½ tablespoon lemon pepper seasoning

Directions

1. Preheat the oven to 3750F and grease a baking tray.
2. Mix together cod fillets, vinegar, lemon pepper seasoning, salt and black pepper in a bowl.
3. Marinate for about 3 hours and then arrange on the baking tray.
4. Transfer into the oven and bake for about 30 minutes.
5. Remove from the oven and serve with herbed butter.

Nutrition Amount per serving

Calories 234

Total Fat 11.8g 15%

Saturated Fat 2.4g 12%

Cholesterol 77mg 26%

Sodium 119mg 5%

Total Carbohydrate 0.4g 0%

Dietary Fiber 0g 0%

Total Sugars 0.1g

Protein 31.5g

Cod Coconut Curry

Serves: 6

Prep Time: 35 mins

Ingredients

- 1 onion, chopped
- 2 pounds cod
- 1 cup dry coconut, chopped
- Salt and black pepper, to taste
- 1 cup fresh lemon juice

Directions

1. Put the cod along with all other ingredients in a pressure cooker.
2. Add 2 cups of water and cover the lid.
3. Cook on High Pressure for about 25 minutes and naturally release the pressure.
4. Open the lid and dish out the curry to serve hot.

Nutrition Amount per serving

Calories 223

Total Fat 6.1g 8%

Saturated Fat 4.5g 23%

Cholesterol 83mg 28%

Sodium 129mg 6%

Total Carbohydrate 4.6g 2%

Dietary Fiber 1.8g 6%

Total Sugars 2.5g

Protein 35.5g

Garlic Shrimp with Goat Cheese

Serves: 4

Prep Time: 30 mins

Ingredients

- 4 tablespoons herbed butter
- Salt and black pepper, to taste
- 1 pound large raw shrimp
- 4 ounces goat cheese
- 4 garlic cloves, chopped

Directions

1. Preheat the oven to 3750F and grease a baking dish.
2. Mix together herbed butter, garlic, raw shrimp, salt and black pepper in a bowl.
3. Put the marinated shrimp on the baking dish and top with the shredded cheese.
4. Place in the oven and bake for about 25 minutes.
5. Take the shrimp out and serve hot.

Nutrition Amount per serving

Calories 294

Total Fat 15g 19%

Saturated Fat 8.9g 44%

Cholesterol 266mg 89%

Sodium 392mg 17%

Total Carbohydrate 2.1g 1%

Dietary Fiber 0.1g 0%

Total Sugars 0.8g

Protein 35.8g

Grain Free Salmon Bread

Serves: 6

Prep Time: 35 mins

Ingredients

- ½ cup olive oil
- ¼ teaspoon baking soda
- ½ cup coconut milk
- 2 pounds salmon, steamed and shredded
- 2 pastured eggs

Directions

1. Preheat the oven to 3750F and grease a baking dish with olive oil.
2. Mix together coconut milk, eggs, baking soda and salmon in a bowl.
3. Pour the batter of salmon bread in the baking dish and transfer into the oven.
4. Bake for about 20 minutes and remove from the oven to serve hot.

Nutrition Amount per serving

Calories 413

Total Fat 32.4g 42%

Saturated Fat 8.5g 42%

Cholesterol 138mg 46%

Sodium 143mg 6%

Total Carbohydrate 1.5g 1%

Dietary Fiber 0.4g 2%

Total Sugars 0.7g

Protein 31.8g

Garlic Parmesan Cod

Serves: 6

Prep Time: 35 mins

Ingredients

- 1 tablespoon extra-virgin olive oil
- 1 (2½) pound cod fillet
- ¼ cup parmesan cheese, finely grated
- Salt and black pepper, to taste
- 5 garlic cloves, minced

Directions

1. Preheat the oven to 4000F and grease a baking dish with cooking spray.
2. Mix together olive oil, garlic, parmesan cheese, salt and black pepper in a bowl.
3. Marinate the cod fillets in this mixture for about 1 hour.
4. Transfer to the baking dish and cover with foil.
5. Place in the oven and bake for about 20 minutes.
6. Remove from the oven and serve warm.

Nutrition Amount per serving

Calories 139

Total Fat 8g 10%

Saturated Fat 1.7g 8%

Cholesterol 37mg 12%

Sodium 77mg 3%

Total Carbohydrate 1g 0%

Dietary Fiber 0.1g 0%

Total Sugars 0g

Protein 16.3g

VEGAN AND VEGETARIAN

Lemon Cream Bok Choy

Serves: 4

Prep Time: 45 mins

Ingredients

- 28 oz. bok choy
- 1 large lemon, juice and zest
- ¾ cup heavy whipping cream
- 1 cup parmesan cheese, freshly grated
- 1 teaspoon black pepper

Directions

1. Preheat the oven to 3500F and lightly grease a baking dish.
2. Pour the cream over the bok choy evenly and drizzle with the lemon juice.
3. Mix well and transfer to the baking dish.
4. Top with parmesan cheese, lemon zest and black pepper and place in the oven.
5. Bake for about 30 minutes until lightly browned and remove from the oven to serve hot.

Nutrition Amount per serving

Calories 199

Total Fat 14.8g 19%

Saturated Fat 9.3g 46%

Cholesterol 51mg 17%

Sodium 398mg 17%

Total Carbohydrate 7.7g 3%

Dietary Fiber 2.5g 9%

Total Sugars 2.7g

Protein 12.7g

Butter Fried Green Cabbage

Serves: 4

Prep Time: 30 mins

Ingredients

- 3 oz. butter
- Salt and black pepper, to taste
- 25 oz. green cabbage, shredded
- 1 tablespoon basil
- ¼ teaspoon red chili flakes

Directions

1. Heat butter in a large skillet over medium heat and add cabbage.
2. Sauté for about 15 minutes, stirring occasionally, until the cabbage is golden brown.
3. Stir in basil, red chili flakes, salt and black pepper and cook for about 3 minutes.
4. Dish out to a bowl and serve hot.

Nutrition Amount per serving

Calories 197

Total Fat 17.4g 22%

Saturated Fat 11g 55%

Cholesterol 46mg 15%

Sodium 301mg 13%

Total Carbohydrate 10.3g 4%

Dietary Fiber 4.5g 16%

Total Sugars 5.7gProtein 2.5g

Broccoli and Cheese

Serves: 4

Prep Time: 20 mins

Ingredients

- 5½ oz. cheddar cheese, shredded
- 23 oz. broccoli, chopped
- 2 oz. butter
- Salt and black pepper, to taste
- 4 tablespoons sour cream

Directions

1. Heat butter in a large skillet over medium high heat and add broccoli, salt and black pepper.
2. Cook for about 5 minutes and stir in the sour cream and cheddar cheese.
3. Cover with lid and cook for about 8 minutes on medium low heat.
4. Dish out to a bowl and serve hot.

Nutrition Amount per serving

Calories 340

Total Fat 27.5g 35%

Saturated Fat 17.1g 85%

Cholesterol 77mg 26%

Sodium 384mg 17%

Total Carbohydrate 11.9g 4%

Dietary Fiber 4.3g 15%

Total Sugars 3g Protein 14.8g

Broccoli Gratin

Serves: 4

Prep Time: 35 mins

Ingredients

- 2 oz. salted butter, for frying
- 5 oz. parmesan cheese, shredded
- 20 oz. broccoli, in florets
- 2 tablespoons Dijon mustard
- ¾ cup crème fraiche

Directions

1. Preheat the oven to 4000F and grease a baking dish lightly.
2. Heat half the butter in a pan on medium low heat and add chopped broccoli.
3. Sauté for about 5 minutes and transfer to the baking dish.
4. Mix the rest of the butter with Dijon mustard and crème fraiche.
5. Pour this mixture in the baking dish and top with parmesan cheese.
6. Transfer to the oven and bake for about 18 minutes.
7. Dish out to a bowl and serve hot.

Nutrition Amount per serving

Calories 338

Total Fat 27.4g 35%

Saturated Fat 12.4g 62%

Cholesterol 56mg 19%

Sodium 546mg 24%

Total Carbohydrate 11.1g 4%

Dietary Fiber 4g 14%

Total Sugars 2.5g

Protein 16.2g

Baked Mini Bell Peppers

Serves: 4

Prep Time: 30 mins

Ingredients

- 1 oz. chorizo, air dried and thinly sliced
- 8 oz. mini bell peppers, sliced lengthwise
- 8 oz. cream cheese
- 1 cup cheddar cheese, shredded
- 1 tablespoon mild chipotle paste

Directions

2. Preheat the oven to 4000F and grease a large baking dish.
3. Mix together cream cheese, chipotle paste, bell peppers and chorizo in a small bowl.
4. Stir the mixture until smooth and transfer to the baking dish.
5. Top with cheddar cheese and place in the oven.
6. Bake for about 20 minutes until the cheese is golden brown and dish onto a platter.

Nutrition Amount per serving

Calories 364

Total Fat 31.9g 41% Saturated Fat 19.4g 97%

Cholesterol 98mg 33%

Sodium 491mg 21%

Total Carbohydrate 6g 2%
Dietary Fiber 0.7g 2% Total Sugars 2.9g

Protein 13.8g

CHICKEN AND POULTRY RECIPES

Turkey with Cream Cheese Sauce

Serves: 4 Prep Time: 30 mins

Ingredients

- 20 oz. turkey breast
- 2 tablespoons butter
- 2 cups heavy whipping cream
- Salt and black pepper, to taste
- 7 oz. cream cheese

Directions

1. Season the turkey generously with salt and black pepper.
2. Heat butter in a skillet over medium heat and cook turkey for about 5 minutes on each side.
3. Stir in the heavy whipping cream and cream cheese.
4. Cover the skillet and cook for about 15 minutes on medium low heat.
5. Dish out to serve hot.

Nutrition Amount per serving

Calories 386

Total Fat 31.7g 41%

Saturated Fat 19.2g 96%

Cholesterol 142mg 47%

Sodium 1100mg 48%

Total Carbohydrate 6g 2%

Dietary Fiber 0.5g 2%

Total Sugars 3.4g

Protein 19.5g

Keto Pesto Chicken Casserole

Serves: 3

Prep Time: 45 mins

Ingredients

- 1½ pounds boneless chicken thighs, cut into bite sized pieces
- Salt and black pepper, to taste
- 2 tablespoons butter
- 3 oz. green pesto
- 5 oz. feta cheese, diced

Directions

1. Preheat the oven to 400 F and grease a baking dish.
2. Season the chicken with salt and black pepper.
3. Heat butter in a skillet over medium heat and cook chicken for about 5 minutes on each side.
4. Dish out in the greased baking dish and add feta cheese and pesto.
5. Transfer the baking dish to the oven and bake for about 30 minutes.
6. Remove from the oven and serve hot.

Nutrition Amount per serving

Calories 438

Total Fat 30.4g 39%

Saturated Fat 11g 55%

Cholesterol 190mg 63%

Sodium 587mg 26%

Total Carbohydrate 1.7g 1%

Dietary Fiber 0g 0%

Total Sugars 1.5g

Protein 39.3g

Italian Turkey

Serves: 6

Prep Time: 25 mins

Ingredients

- 1½ cups Italian dressing
- Salt and black pepper, to taste
- 2 tablespoons butter
- 1 (2 pound) bone-in turkey breast
- 2 garlic cloves, minced

Directions

1. Preheat the oven to 3500F and grease a baking dish with butter.
2. Mix together minced garlic cloves, salt and black pepper and rub the turkey breast with this mixture.
3. Arrange turkey breast in the baking dish and top evenly with Italian dressing.
4. Bake for about 2 hours, coating with pan juices occasionally.
5. Dish out and serve immediately.

Nutrition Amount per serving

Calories 464

Total Fat 31.3g 40%

Saturated Fat 7.8g 39%

Cholesterol 144mg 48%

Sodium 234mg 10%

Total Carbohydrate 6.5g 2%

Dietary Fiber 0g 0%

Total Sugars 4.9g

Protein 32.7g

Caprese Chicken

Serves: 4

Prep Time: 30 mins

Ingredients

- 1 pound chicken breasts, boneless and skinless
- ¼ cup balsamic vinegar
- 1 tablespoon extra-virgin olive oil
- Kosher salt and black pepper, to taste
- 4 mozzarella cheese slices

Directions

1. Season the chicken with salt and black pepper.
2. Heat olive oil in a skillet over medium heat and cook chicken for about 5 minutes on each side.
3. Stir in the balsamic vinegar and cook for about 2 minutes.
4. Add mozzarella cheese slices and cook for about 2 minutes until melted.
5. Dish out in a plate and serve hot.

Nutrition Amount per serving

Calories 329

Total Fat 16.9g 22%

Saturated Fat 5.8g 29%

Cholesterol 116mg 39%

Sodium 268mg 12%

Total Carbohydrate 1.1g 0%

Dietary Fiber 0g 0%

Total Sugars 0.1g

Protein 40.8g

Roasted Chicken with Herbed Butter

Serves: 6

Prep Time: 30 mins

Ingredients

- 1 tablespoon garlic paste
- 6 chicken legs
- 4 cups water
- Salt, to taste
- 4 tablespoons herbed butter

Directions

1. Season the chicken legs with salt and mix with garlic paste.
2. Put a rack in an electric pressure cooker and add water.
3. Place the marinated pieces of chicken on the rack and lock the lid.
4. Cook on high pressure for about 15 minutes.
5. Naturally release the pressure and dish out in a platter.
6. Spread herbed butter on the chicken legs and serve.

Nutrition Amount per serving

Calories 304

Total Fat 12.7g 16%

Saturated Fat 3.8g 19%

Cholesterol 137mg 46%

Sodium 177mg 8%

Total Carbohydrate 0.7g 0%

Dietary Fiber 0g 0%

Total Sugars 0.1g

Protein 44g

Chicken Enchiladas

Serves: 2

Prep Time: 25 mins

Ingredients

- 2 ounces chicken, shredded
- ½ tablespoon olive oil
- 2 ounces shiitake mushrooms, chopped
- Sea salt and black pepper, to taste
- ½ teaspoon apple cider vinegar

Directions

1. Heat olive oil in a skillet and add mushrooms.
2. Sauté for about 30 seconds and stir in chicken.
3. Cook for about 2 minutes and pour in apple cider vinegar.
4. Season with sea salt and black pepper and cover the lid.
5. Cook for about 20 minutes on medium low heat.
6. Dish out and serve hot.

Nutrition Amount per serving

Calories 88

Total Fat 4.4g 6%

Saturated Fat 0.8g 4%

Cholesterol 22mg 7%

Sodium 86mg 4%

Total Carbohydrate 3.9g 1%

Dietary Fiber 0.6g 2%

Total Sugars 1g

Protein 8.7g

Turkey Balls

Serves: 6

Prep Time: 35 mins

Ingredients

- 1 cup broccoli, chopped
- 1 pound turkey, boiled and chopped
- 2 teaspoons ginger-garlic paste
- Salt and lemon pepper seasoning, to taste
- ½ cup olive oil

Directions

1. Preheat the oven to 3600F and grease a baking tray.
2. Mix together turkey, olive oil, broccoli, ginger-garlic paste, salt and lemon pepper seasoning in a bowl.
3. Make small balls out of this mixture and arrange on the baking tray.
4. Transfer to the oven and bake for about 20 minutes.
5. Remove from the oven and serve with the dip of your choice.

Nutrition Amount per serving

Calories 275

Total Fat 20.1g 26%

Saturated Fat 3g 15%

Cholesterol 58mg 19%

Sodium 53mg 2%

Total Carbohydrate 1.5g 1%

Dietary Fiber 0.4g 1%

Total Sugars 0.3g

Protein 22.4g

Chicken Zucchini Cutlets

Serves: 6

Prep Time: 20 mins

Ingredients

- 3 zucchinis, boiled and mashed
- 3 tablespoons lemon pepper seasoning
- ½ pound chicken, boiled and chopped
- ½ cup avocado oil
- Salt and black pepper, to taste

Directions

1. Mix together chicken, zucchinis, lemon pepper seasoning, salt and black pepper in a bowl.
2. Make cutlets out of this mixture and set aside.
3. Heat avocado oil in a pan and put the cutlets in it.
4. Fry for about 2-3 minutes on each side and dish out to serve.

Nutrition Amount per serving

Calories 106

Total Fat 3.8g 5%

Saturated Fat 0.9g 4%

Cholesterol 29mg 10%

Sodium 36mg 2%

Total Carbohydrate 6.4g 2%

Dietary Fiber 2.8g 10%

Total Sugars 1.8g

Protein 12.7g

Low Carb Chicken Nuggets

Serves: 6

Prep Time: 25 mins Ingredients

- ¼ cup mayonnaise
- 2 medium chicken breasts
- 1 cup blanched almond flour
- 2 tablespoons olive oil
- Sea salt and black pepper, to taste

Directions

1. Put the chicken in the salted water for about 10 minutes.
2. Drain it and cut the chicken into nugget sized pieces.
3. Put mayonnaise in one bowl and mix almond flour, sea salt and black pepper in another bowl.
4. Coat each chicken nugget with mayonnaise and dredge in the almond flour mixture.
5. Heat oil over medium high heat in a skillet and add chicken nuggets in a single layer.
6. Cook for about 3 minutes per side until golden and dish out to serve.

Nutrition Amount per serving

Calories 283

Total Fat 20.4g 26%

Saturated Fat 2.8g 14%

Cholesterol 46mg 15%

Sodium 118mg 5%

Total Carbohydrate 6.3g 2%

Dietary Fiber 2g 7%

Total Sugars 0.6g

Protein 18.2g

CPSIA information can be obtained
at www.ICGtesting.com
Printed in the USA
LVHW020356010221
677957LV00006BA/231